JUICING

FOR

MIGRAINE RELIEF

30 Natural and Nutritional Recipe for Severe Headache

Dr. Lauren C. Riley

TABLE OF CONTENT

INTRODUCTION

Are you tired of the throbbing pain and debilitating symptoms of migraines? Do you yearn for a natural, holistic approach to managing this chronic condition that plagues your everyday life? If so, you've come to the correct place.. Welcome to a transformative journey that will introduce you to the extraordinary world of juicing and its remarkable benefits for migraine sufferers.

In this book, we will delve deep into the art and science of juicing, exploring its potential to alleviate the excruciating pain and discomfort caused by migraines. But beyond simply providing relief, we will uncover the multitude of health benefits that juicing offers, providing you with a comprehensive understanding of how this practice can improve your overall well-being.

Migraine, a neurological disorder characterized by intense headaches, sensory disturbances, and other associated symptoms, affects millions of people worldwide. Traditional treatments often involve prescription medications that come with a host of side effects and limitations.

The desire for a more natural and sustainable solution has led many individuals on a quest to explore alternative therapies, ultimately leading them to the realm of juicing.

Juicing, the process of extracting the nutrient-rich juices from fruits and vegetables, has gained immense popularity in recent years for its ability to nourish the body at a cellular level. These vibrant elixirs, bursting with vitamins, minerals, antioxidants, and other essential compounds, have the power to revitalize and heal the body from within. It is this remarkable potential that makes juicing an invaluable tool in the management of migraines.

Here are *30 juicing recipes* specifically designed to target migraines. Each recipe includes the ingredients, preparation method, and nutritional value to help you understand the benefits they offer. Remember to use fresh, organic ingredients whenever possible for optimal results.

1. Migraine Buster

Ingredients:

2 apples

2 celery stalks

1 cucumber

1-inch piece of ginger

Preparation:

Wash all the ingredients thoroughly.

Core the apples and cut them into chunks.

Slice the celery stalks, cucumber, and ginger.

Pass all the ingredients through a juicer.

Stir well and serve immediately.

This recipe combines the hydrating properties of cucumber, the anti-inflammatory benefits of ginger, and the antioxidant-rich apples to provide relief from migraines while boosting your immune system.

2. Green Zing

Ingredients:

2 cups spinach

1 cucumber

1 green apple

1 lemon

Preparation:

Rinse the spinach leaves.

Peel and slice the cucumber.

Core and chop the green apple.

Juice the spinach, cucumber, green apple, and lemon.

Mix well and serve chilled.

This recipe is packed with magnesium from spinach, hydrating properties of cucumber, vitamin C from lemon, and the soothing effects of green apple. It helps reduce inflammation and supports overall brain health.

3. Citrus Bliss

Ingredients:

2 oranges

1 grapefruit

1-inch piece of turmeric

Preparation:

Peel and separate the oranges and grapefruit into sections.

Cut the turmeric into smaller pieces.

Run the oranges, grapefruit, and turmeric through a juicer.

Stir well and enjoy.

Nutritional Value:

Oranges and grapefruits are rich in vitamin C, while turmeric contains curcumin, a powerful anti-inflammatory compound. This recipe helps reduce inflammation, relieve pain, and boost your immune system.

4. Berry Delight

Ingredients:

1 cup strawberries

1 cup blueberries

1 cup raspberries

1 cup coconut water

Preparation:

Wash all the berries thoroughly.

Place the berries in a blender or juicer.

Add the coconut water.

Blend until smooth.

Serve over ice.

Nutritional Value:

Berries are packed with antioxidants, vitamins, and minerals that support brain health. This recipe provides a refreshing and nourishing blend to reduce inflammation and promote overall well-being.

5. Pineapple Mint Refresher

Ingredients:

1 cup pineapple chunks

Handful of fresh mint leaves

1 lime

1 teaspoon honey (optional)

Preparation:

Peel and chop the pineapple.

Rinse the mint leaves.

Squeeze the juice from the lime.

Combine pineapple, mint leaves, lime juice, and honey (if desired) in a blender.

Blend until smooth.

Pour into a glass and serve chilled.

Pineapple contains bromelain, an enzyme known for its anti-inflammatory properties, while mint provides a soothing effect. This refreshing recipe helps reduce migraines and provides a burst of tropical flavors.

6. Carrot Ginger Elixir

Ingredients:

3 carrots

1-inch piece of ginger

1 orange

Preparation:

Wash and peel the carrots.

Peel and slice the ginger.

Peel and separate the orange into sections.

Juice the carrots, ginger, and orange.

Mix well and serve over ice.

Carrots are rich in beta-carotene, a powerful antioxidant that helps reduce inflammation and protect against oxidative stress. Ginger adds a spicy kick and has anti-inflammatory properties, while oranges provide a boost of vitamin C. This elixir not only aids in migraine relief but also supports healthy digestion and immune function.

7. Beetroot Bliss

Ingredients:

1 beetroot

2 carrots

1 apple

1 lemon

Preparation:

Wash and peel the beetroot, carrots, and apple.

Cut them into chunks.

Juice the beetroot, carrots, apple, and lemon.

Stir well and serve chilled.

Beetroot is a nutritional powerhouse, containing compounds that help dilate blood vessels, reduce inflammation, and improve blood flow to the brain. Carrots and apples provide additional vitamins and minerals, while lemon adds a refreshing twist. This recipe promotes circulation and helps alleviate migraines.

8. Cooling Cucumber

Ingredients:

2 cucumbers

1 cup fresh mint leaves

1 lime

Preparation:

Wash the cucumbers and cut them into chunks.

Rinse the mint leaves.

Squeeze the juice from the lime.

Add the cucumbers, mint leaves, and lime juice to a blender.

Blend until smooth.

Serve chilled.

Nutritional Value:

Cucumbers are hydrating and cooling, which can be beneficial for migraines. Mint offers a soothing effect, while lime provides a refreshing zing. This recipe hydrates and cools the body, helping to alleviate migraine symptoms.

9. Ginger Turmeric Tonic

Ingredients:

1-inch piece of ginger

1-inch piece of turmeric

2 carrots

1 orange

Preparation:

Peel and slice the ginger and turmeric.

Wash and peel the carrots.

Peel and separate the orange into sections.

Juice the ginger, turmeric, carrots, and orange.

Mix well and serve over ice.

Ginger and turmeric both have potent anti-inflammatory properties that can help reduce migraines. Carrots and oranges provide additional vitamins and antioxidants. This tonic is a powerful elixir for migraine relief and overall wellness.

10. Greens and Berries Blend

Ingredients:

2 cups kale

1 cup spinach

1 cup mixed berries (strawberries, blueberries, raspberries)

1 banana

1 cup almond milk

Wash the kale and spinach leaves.

Hull the strawberries.

Place all the ingredients in a blender.

Blend until smooth.

Pour into a glass and serve chilled.

Nutritional Value:

Kale and spinach are rich in magnesium and other essential nutrients that can help prevent migraines. Berries provide antioxidants, while banana adds creaminess and sweetness. This nutrient-packed blend supports brain health and offers a delicious way to consume greens.

11. Tangy Mango Twist

Ingredients:

1 ripe mango

1 orange

1 lime

Handful of fresh cilantro

Preparation:

Peel and chop the mango.

Squeeze the juice from the orange and lime.

Rinse the cilantro.

Nutritional Value:

Mangoes are rich in vitamins A and C, while oranges and lime provide additional vitamin C. Cilantro adds a unique flavor and offers detox properties. This tangy and refreshing juice provides a burst of tropical flavors while supporting migraine relief and overall health.

12. Blueberry Lavender Soother

Ingredients:

1 cup blueberries

1 cup almond milk

1 teaspoon dried lavender buds

1 tablespoon honey (optional)

Preparation:

Rinse the blueberries.

In a small saucepan, gently warm the almond milk over low heat.

Add the dried lavender buds to the warm almond milk and let steep for 5 minutes.

Strain the almond milk to remove the lavender buds.

In a blender, combine the blueberries, lavender-infused almond milk, and honey (if desired).

Blend until smooth.

Serve chilled.

Nutritional Value:

Blueberries are rich in antioxidants and have anti-inflammatory properties that can help reduce migraines. Lavender has a calming effect on the nervous system, promoting relaxation and stress reduction. This soothing blend is perfect for easing migraine symptoms and promoting restful sleep.

13. Watermelon Mint Cooler

Ingredients:

2 cups watermelon cubes

Handful of fresh mint leaves

Juice of 1 lime

Preparation:

Remove the seeds from the watermelon cubes.

Rinse the mint leaves.

Squeeze the juice from the lime.

In a blender, combine the watermelon cubes, mint leaves, and lime juice.

Blend until smooth.

Serve over ice.

Nutritional Value:

Watermelon is incredibly hydrating, and its high water content can help alleviate dehydration-induced migraines. Mint adds a refreshing flavor and aids digestion, while lime provides a burst of citrusy tang. This cooling and hydrating cooler is perfect for hot summer days and migraine relief.

14. Spinach Pineapple Punch

Ingredients:

2 cups spinach

1 cup pineapple chunks

1 banana

1 cup coconut water

Preparation:

Wash the spinach leaves.

Peel and chop the pineapple.

Peel the banana.

In a blender, combine the spinach, pineapple chunks, banana, and coconut water.

Blend until smooth.

Serve chilled.

Spinach is rich in magnesium and other essential nutrients that can help prevent migraines. Pineapple adds a tropical sweetness and contains bromelain, an enzyme with anti-inflammatory properties. Banana adds creaminess and potassium, while coconut water provides electrolytes and hydration. This punch is a nutrient-packed and delicious way to support migraine relief and overall health.

15. Kiwi Ginger Refresher

Ingredients:

2 kiwis

1-inch piece of ginger

Juice of 1 lemon

1 tablespoon honey (optional)

Preparation:

Peel and chop the kiwis.

Peel and slice the ginger.

Squeeze the juice from the lemon.

In a blender, combine the kiwis, ginger, lemon juice, and honey (if desired).

Blend until smooth.

Serve chilled.

Nutritional Value:

Kiwi is rich in vitamin C and other antioxidants that can help reduce inflammation and support immune health. Ginger adds a spicy kick and has anti-inflammatory properties, while lemon provides a citrusy tang. This refreshing refresher aids in migraine relief and provides a boost of nutrients.

16. Turmeric Pineapple Elixir

Ingredients:

1 cup pineapple chunks

1 teaspoon turmeric powder

1 cup coconut water

Juice of 1 lime

Preparation:

Peel and chop the pineapple.

In a blender, combine the pineapple chunks, turmeric powder, coconut water, and lime juice

Blend until smooth.

Serve over ice.

Nutritional Value:

Pineapple contains bromelain, an enzyme with anti-inflammatory properties, while turmeric is renowned for its powerful anti-inflammatory compound, curcumin. Coconut water provides hydration and electrolytes, and lime adds a refreshing zing. This elixir is a potent anti-inflammatory blend that aids in migraine relief and promotes overall well-being.

17. Carrot Berry Boost

Ingredients:

2 carrots

1 cup mixed berries (strawberries, blueberries, raspberries)

1 orange

1 tablespoon chia seeds

Preparation:

Wash and peel the carrots.

Rinse the berries.

Peel and separate the orange into sections.

Juice the carrots, berries, and orange.

Stir in the chia seeds.

Let it sit for a few minutes to allow the chia seeds to absorb some liquid.

Mix well and serve chilled.

Nutritional Value:

Carrots are packed with nutrients and antioxidants that support brain health. Berries provide an abundance of antioxidants, while oranges add a tangy sweetness. Chia seeds offer omega-3 fatty acids, fiber, and additional nutrients. This nutrient-rich blend boosts energy, aids in migraine relief, and promotes a healthy digestive system.

18. Minty Melon Medley

Ingredients:

2 cups cubed honeydew melon

Handful of fresh mint leaves

Juice of 1 lime

1 teaspoon honey (optional)

Preparation:

Cut the honeydew melon into cubes.

Rinse the mint leaves.

Squeeze the juice from the lime.

In a blender, combine the honeydew melon cubes, mint leaves, lime juice, and honey (if desired).

Blend until smooth.

Serve chilled.

Nutritional Value:

Honeydew melon is hydrating and rich in vitamins and minerals, while mint provides a refreshing flavor and aids digestion. Lime adds a tangy twist and boosts vitamin C content. This medley is perfect for soothing migraines and keeping you cool and hydrated.

19. Kale Apple Zinger

Ingredients:

2 cups kale

2 green apples

1 cucumber

1-inch piece of ginger

Preparation:

Wash the kale leaves.

Core and chop the green apples.

Slice the cucumber.

Peel and slice the ginger.

Pass the kale, green apples, cucumber, and ginger through a juicer.

Stir well and serve immediately.

Kale is packed with vitamins, minerals, and antioxidants that support brain health. Green apples provide a burst of flavor and additional nutrients, while cucumber hydrates and ginger adds a zingy kick. This zinger juice aids in reducing inflammation and supports overall well-being.

20. Citrus Carrot Splash

Ingredients:

3 carrots

1 orange

1 grapefruit

1 lemon

Preparation:

Wash and peel the carrots.

Peel and separate the orange and grapefruit into sections.

Squeeze the juice from the lemon.

Juice the carrots, orange, grapefruit, and lemon.

Mix well and serve over ice.

Carrots are rich in beta-carotene and other essential nutrients that support brain health. Oranges, grapefruits, and lemons are high in vitamin C, which can help reduce inflammation and support immune health. This refreshing citrus blend provides a burst of vitamins and antioxidants, aiding in migraine relief and promoting overall wellness.

21. Cooling Cabbage Blend

Ingredients:

2 cups green cabbage

1 cucumber

1 green apple

Juice of 1 lemon

Preparation:

Wash the cabbage leaves.

Slice the cucumber.

Core and chop the green apple.

Squeeze the juice from the lemon.

In a blender, combine the cabbage leaves, cucumber, green apple, and lemon juice.

Blend until smooth.

Serve chilled.

Green cabbage is rich in antioxidants and anti-inflammatory compounds that can help reduce migraines. Cucumber provides hydration, while green apple adds a touch of sweetness. Lemon adds a citrusy tang and boosts the vitamin C content.

This cooling blend supports migraine relief and promotes a healthy inflammatory response.

22. Papaya Ginger Elixir

Ingredients:

1 cup ripe papaya chunks

1-inch piece of ginger

Juice of 1 lime

1 tablespoon honey (optional)

Preparation:

Peel and chop the papaya.

Peel and slice the ginger.

Squeeze the juice from the lime.

In a blender, combine the papaya chunks, ginger, lime juice, and honey (if desired).

Blend until smooth.

Serve over ice.

Nutritional Value:

Papaya is rich in enzymes, vitamins, and antioxidants that support digestion and reduce inflammation. Ginger adds a spicy kick and aids in migraine relief, while lime provides a tangy twist. This tropical elixir is refreshing and beneficial for migraines and overall well-being.

23. Mixed Greens Detox

Ingredients:

1 cup spinach

1 cup kale

1 cup parsley

1 cucumber

Juice of 1 lemon

Preparation:

Wash the spinach, kale, and parsley leaves.

Slice the cucumber.

Squeeze the juice from the lemon.

In a juicer or blender, combine the spinach, kale, parsley, cucumber, and lemon juice.

Blend until smooth.

Serve chilled.

Nutritional Value:

This detoxifying blend combines the cleansing properties of spinach, kale, and parsley. Cucumber adds hydration and additional detoxification benefits, while lemon provides a burst of vitamin C and aids digestion. This green elixir helps eliminate toxins and supports overall wellness.

24. Pineapple Ginger Zest

Ingredients:

1 cup pineapple chunks

1-inch piece of ginger

Handful of fresh basil leaves

Juice of 1 lime

Preparation:

Peel and chop the pineapple.

Peel and slice the ginger.

Rinse the basil leaves.

Squeeze the juice from the lime.

In a blender, combine the pineapple chunks, ginger, basil leaves, and lime juice.

Blend until smooth.

Serve chilled.

Pineapple contains bromelain, an enzyme that helps reduce inflammation and supports digestion. Ginger adds a zingy kick and aids in migraine relief, while basil provides a refreshing flavor. Lime adds a citrusy twist and boosts the vitamin C content. This zesty blend is a refreshing way to alleviate migraines and support overall well-being.

25. Strawberry Mint Splash

Ingredients:

1 cup strawberries

Handful of fresh mint leaves

1 cup coconut water

Juice of 1 lemon

Preparation:

Hull the strawberries.

Rinse the mint leaves.

In a blender, combine the strawberries, mint leaves, coconut water, and lemon juice.

Blend until smooth.

Serve over ice.

Nutritional Value:

Strawberries are rich in antioxidants and have anti-inflammatory properties that can help reduce migraines. Mint adds a refreshing flavor and aids digestion, while coconut water provides hydration and electrolytes. Lemon adds a tangy twist and boosts the vitamin C content. This refreshing splash is perfect for soothing migraines and keeping you cool and hydrated.

26. Cucumber Celery Refresher

Ingredients:

1 cucumber

3 stalks of celery

Handful of fresh parsley

Juice of 1 lemon

Preparation:

Wash the cucumber, celery, and parsley.

Slice the cucumber and celery into chunks.

In a juicer or blender, combine the cucumber, celery, parsley, and lemon juice.

Blend until smooth.

Serve chilled.

Nutritional Value:

Cucumber and celery both have high water content, providing hydration and reducing the risk of dehydration-induced migraines. Parsley adds a fresh and herbaceous flavor, while lemon provides a tangy twist and aids digestion. This refreshing refresher is perfect for soothing migraines and replenishing fluids.

27. Mango Turmeric Twist

Ingredients:

1 ripe mango

1 teaspoon turmeric powder

1 cup coconut milk

1 tablespoon honey (optional)

Preparation:

Peel and chop the mango.

In a blender, combine the mango chunks, turmeric powder, coconut milk, and honey (if desired).

Blend until smooth.

Serve chilled.

Nutritional Value:

Mangoes are rich in vitamins A and C, as well as antioxidants that can help reduce inflammation and support immune health. Turmeric adds a warm and earthy flavor and contains curcumin, a compound with potent anti-inflammatory properties. Coconut milk provides a creamy base and offers healthy fats. This twist is a delicious way to enjoy the benefits of turmeric and mango while aiding in migraine relief.

28. Berry Blast Smoothie

Ingredients:

1 cup mixed berries (strawberries, blueberries, raspberries)

1 banana

1 cup almond milk

1 tablespoon flaxseeds

Preparation:

Rinse the berries.

Peel the banana.

In a blender, combine the mixed berries, banana, almond milk, and flaxseeds.

Blend until smooth.

Serve chilled.

Nutritional Value:

Berries are packed with antioxidants and anti-inflammatory compounds that can help reduce migraines. Banana adds creaminess and natural sweetness, while almond milk provides a dairy-free and nutritious base. Flaxseeds offer omega-3 fatty acids and fiber. This berry blast smoothie is a delicious and nutrient-packed option for migraine relief and overall well-being.

29. Ginger Peach Delight

Ingredients:

2 peaches

1-inch piece of ginger

Handful of fresh basil leaves

1 cup coconut water

Preparation:

Peel and slice the peaches.

Peel and slice the ginger.

Rinse the basil leaves.

In a blender, combine the peaches, ginger, basil leaves, and coconut water.

Blend until smooth.

Serve chilled.

Peaches are rich in vitamins and minerals, including potassium, which can help alleviate migraines. Ginger adds a zingy kick and aids in migraine relief, while basil provides a fresh and aromatic flavor. Coconut water adds hydration and electrolytes. This delightful blend combines fruity sweetness with a hint of spice, making it a perfect choice for soothing migraines and refreshing the body.

30. Pineapple Celery Detox

Ingredients:

1 cup pineapple chunks

3 stalks of celery

Handful of fresh cilantro

Juice of 1 lime

Preparation:

Peel and chop the pineapple.

Slice the celery into chunks.

Rinse the cilantro.

Squeeze the juice from the lime.

In a blender, combine the pineapple chunks, celery, cilantro, and lime juice.

Blend until smooth.

Serve chilled.

Nutritional Value:

Pineapple contains bromelain, an enzyme with anti-inflammatory properties, while celery is known for its high water content and detoxifying effects. Cilantro adds a refreshing flavor and aids in detoxification, while lime provides a tangy twist and boosts vitamin C content. This detoxifying blend helps eliminate toxins, hydrates the body, and supports migraine relief.

These 30 juicing recipes offer a variety of delicious options to support migraine relief while providing essential nutrients and hydration. Remember to consult with a healthcare professional if you have any specific dietary concerns or sensitivities. Enjoy these flavorful blends and their potential benefits for overall well-being.

CONCLUSION

Juicing for migraine relief offers a natural and nutritious approach to managing and alleviating migraine symptoms. By incorporating fresh fruits, vegetables, herbs, and spices into your daily routine, you can harness the power of antioxidants, anti-inflammatory compounds, and essential nutrients to support brain health, reduce inflammation, and promote overall well-being.

The 30 juicing recipes provided in this book offer a wide range of flavors and combinations that not only taste delicious but also provide specific benefits for migraine relief. From soothing ginger-infused blends to hydrating cucumber-based elixirs and nutrient-rich green concoctions, these recipes are designed to target inflammation, support digestion, and replenish essential nutrients.

It's important to note that while juicing can be a beneficial addition to your migraine management plan, it's always recommended to consult with a healthcare professional to ensure it aligns with your specific needs and any existing dietary restrictions. Additionally, it's crucial to listen to your body and make adjustments as needed, as everyone's triggers and sensitivities can vary.

Incorporating juicing into your lifestyle goes beyond just addressing the symptoms of migraines. It can also promote overall health and well-being by boosting your intake of vitamins, minerals, antioxidants, and hydration. Remember, a balanced and nutritious diet, along with regular.exercise, adequate sleep, stress management, and a healthy lifestyle, all play a role in managing migraines holistically.

So, grab your juicer, stock up on fresh produce, and embark on a flavorful journey to support your migraine relief. Experiment with the recipes provided in this book, customize them to suit your taste preferences, and discover the ones that work best for you. Cheers to a healthier, happier life with fewer migraines!